ESSENTIAL GUIDE TO XERODERMA PIGMENTSUM

Unlocking the Secrets: A Comprehensive Guide to Xeroderma Pigmentosum Management and Care

DR. CASEY LOREN

DISCLAIMER

This book's content is only meant to be used for general informative purposes. Although the author has taken great care to ensure the content is accurate and thorough, no warranties or assurances on the information's accuracy, correctness, or reliability are provided. It is recommended that readers employ their own judgment and discretion when applying any material found in this book to their particular situation.

The information in this book is not intended to replace professional advice, nor is the author an expert in any of the subjects covered. It is recommended that readers consult with experienced professionals regarding any particular issues or concerns.

Any name that may be mentioned or referred in this book does not imply endorsement, recommendation, or relationship on the part of the author with any person, entity, good, website, or association. These references are made only for informational purposes and are not meant to be taken as recommendations or endorsements.

The information contained in this book may cause readers to suffer loss or damage, for which the author disclaims all obligation and accountability. The only people accountable for the decisions and actions taken by readers using the information presented are themselves.

Any names, characters, companies, locations, activities, occasions, and incidents referenced in this book are either made up or the result of the author's imagination. Any likeness to real people, living or dead, or to real things is entirely coincidental.

This book's content may change at any time, without prior notice, according to the author. The onus is on the reader to verify whether there have been any updates or revisions.

The reader accepts the conditions of this disclaimer by reading this book. Please do not read this book or use its contents if you do not agree to these terms.

Table of Contents

CHAPTER 1

XERODERMA PIGMENTOSUM (XP): AN OVERVIEW

A Comprehensive Overview of Xeroderma Pigmentosum (XP)

Definition and Synopsis

The rare hereditary condition known as Xeroderma Pigmentosum (XP) is typified by an intense sensitivity to ultraviolet (UV) radiation emitted by sunshine. This disorder usually appears in early childhood and increases the risk of skin cancer and other abnormalities because UV light damages DNA, which the body is unable to repair. Since XP is an autosomal recessive disorder, a kid cannot be impacted unless both parents have the faulty gene.

XP's Discovery and History

The first description of XP was given by the Hungarian dermatologist Moritz Kaposi in 1874. He reported that young people with the disorder had a high prevalence of skin cancer and dry, pigmented skin abnormalities. Our knowledge of XP has greatly advanced as a result of research that has revealed the underlying genetic causes and mechanisms of the condition. Understanding the pathogenesis of XP required the identification of the flaw in nucleotide excision repair (NER), a DNA repair mechanism.

Demographics and Prevalence

XP is a very uncommon condition that affects about 1 in 1,000,000 people in Europe and the United States. Nonetheless, it is more widespread in areas like Japan, North Africa, and the Middle East where consanguineous marriages—marriages between closely related people—are more typical. XP is prevalent in all ethnic groups and equally affects men and women.

XP's Genetic Basis

Gene mutations that affect the nucleotide excision repair (NER) pathway, which fixes UV-induced DNA damage, are the cause of XP. At least eight genes—XP-A through XP-G and XP-V, a mutant form—have been linked to XP. Every gene has a distinct function in identifying and removing damaged DNA. These genes' mutations hinder the repair mechanism, which increases the risk of cancer, accumulates DNA damage, and kills cells.

XP Kinds and Classifications

Depending on the particular gene mutation involved, XP is categorized into multiple complementation categories. Among them are:

1. **XP-A**: Neurological problems in a severe degree.

2. **XP-B**: Infrequent, frequently connected to Cockayne syndrome.

3. **XP-C**: Common in the United States; usually not neurologically problematic.

4. **XP-D**: Neurological symptoms may or may not be present.

5. **XP-E**: Infrequent, less severe symptoms.

6. Rare; frequently has a moderate phenotype (**XP-F**).

7. **XP-G**: Cockayne syndrome may coexist with it.

8. **XP-V**: Polymerase eta gene defect resulting in less severe symptoms.

The severity of each type varies according to the particular genetic abnormality.

Clinical Presentation and Symptoms

Extreme sun sensitivity, which frequently results in severe sunburns after little to no sun exposure, is the defining characteristic of XP. Additional signs and symptoms consist of:

- **Skin Changes**: Freckles, dry skin, and altered pigmentation in regions exposed to the sun.

- **Skin Cancer**: Protection against skin malignancies at an early age, including melanoma, squamous cell carcinoma, and basal cell carcinoma.

- **Ocular Problems**: elevated risk of eye malignancies, keratitis, conjunctivitis, and photophobia.

- **Neurological impairments**: Hearing loss, cognitive decline, and coordination impairments are among the progressive neurological concerns that some people may experience.

The Significance of Prompt Diagnosis

XP must be diagnosed as soon as possible to manage the condition and reduce its hazards.

Early detection enables the application of stringent UV protection protocols, which can dramatically lower the risk of skin and ocular malignancies. Genetic testing and counseling can help with early diagnosis and provide families with guidance on how to properly manage the condition.

Effect on Life Quality

The quality of life for those who are affected by XP and their families is significantly impacted. Patients are required to follow strict guidelines for protecting themselves from the sun, such as donning protective clothes, applying high-SPF sunscreen, and avoiding direct sunlight. This may restrict social connections and outdoor activities, which may hurt mental and emotional health. The cost of healthcare is increased by routine checkups with doctors and treatments for skin malignancies and other issues.

XP Myths & Misconceptions

There are a few common misconceptions regarding XP, such as:

Myth: There is a contagious XP.

Fact: XP is a hereditary disorder that cannot be passed from one person to another.

- **Myth**: Neurological problems affect every XP patient.

Fact: Not all varieties of XP cause neurological issues; some only have skin-related symptoms.

- **Myth**: In the shade, you don't need to wear sunscreen.

Fact: Protection is always required since UV rays can reflect off surfaces and pass through clouds.

Objective and Coverage of the Guide

This guide's main goal is to give patients a thorough understanding of Xeroderma Pigmentosum, including everything from the condition's clinical manifestation and genetic foundation to its effects on their quality of life. By educating patients, families, medical professionals, and the general public about XP, this guide hopes to raise awareness and understanding of this uncommon condition. Through providing comprehensive analyses and dispelling prevalent misconceptions, this manual aims to facilitate enhanced supervision and treatment of XP patients.

CHAPTER 2

XP'S GENETIC AND MOLECULAR FOUNDATION

The Molecular and Genetic Foundations of Xeroderma Pigmentosum (XP)

Extreme sensitivity to ultraviolet (UV) rays from sunshine is the hallmark of Xeroderma Pigmentosum (XP), a rare genetic condition that increases the risk of skin cancer and other abnormalities. It is essential to comprehend the genetic and molecular causes of XP to diagnose, treat, and possibly even create future treatments for this illness.

Mechanisms of DNA Repair

To preserve genomic stability and stop mutations that can cause illnesses like cancer, DNA repair systems are crucial. The main flaw in XP is related to DNA repair, namely with the machinery involved in repairing UV-induced damage. The accumulation of mutations brought on by this incapacity to repair DNA damage causes the clinical signs and symptoms of XP.

Nucleotide Excision Repair's (NER) Function

The crucial DNA repair process that is faulty in XP is Nucleotide Excision Repair (NER). NER is in charge of finding and eliminating a variety of DNA lesions, including ones brought on by UV light and including 6-4 photoproducts and cyclobutane pyrimidine dimers (CPDs). There are multiple steps in the NER process:

1. **Damage Recognition**: Proteins attach to the DNA lesion after recognizing it.

2. **Excision**: A brief section of single-stranded DNA containing the lesion is removed by endonucleases.

3. **DNA Synthesis**: Using the intact strand as a template, DNA polymerase fills in the missing sequence.

4. **Ligation**: The newly synthesized DNA is sealed into the preexisting strand by DNA ligase.

Genes Connected to XP

Mutations in multiple NER pathway-related genes are linked to XP. Among these genes are:

- **XPA**: Contributes to the development of repair complexes and damage identification.

A helicase called **XPB (ERCC3)** unwinds the DNA surrounding the damaged site.

- **XPC**: Commences global genome NER upon detecting DNA damage.

- **XPD (ERCC2)**: An important helicase that unwinds DNA in the course of repair.

- **XPE (DDB2)**: Catches UV-damaged DNA and starts the healing process.

An endonuclease that cuts close to the DNA lesion is **XPF (ERCC4)**.

An endonuclease that also incises DNA close to the damage is **XPG (ERCC5)**.

Types of Mutations in XP Genes

XP gene mutations can take many different forms, such as:

Missense, nonsense, and splice site mutations can result from **point mutations**, which are single nucleotide alterations.

- **Insertions/Deletions (indels)**: Modifications of any size that may interfere with the reading frame of a gene.

- **Significant deletions**: Complete exons or even more extensive genomic regions absent.

- **Complex rearrangements**: Chromosome structural alterations that impact gene function.

The Cellular Pathophysiology of XP

The following outcomes occur at the cellular level when UV-induced DNA damage is not repaired:

- **Agglomeration of DNA mutations**: Raises the danger of developing skin cancer and other cancers.

Cellular apoptosis: Cells that have been damaged may die according to a set schedule.

- **Impaired transcription and replication**: Impairs the viability and general function of the cell.

- **Persistent inflammation**: May be a factor in the development of cancer and abnormalities of the skin.

Patterns of Inheritance

Because XP has an autosomal recessive inheritance pattern, a person must inherit two faulty copies of the XP gene—one from each parent—to develop the illness. Carriers, who have one faulty allele and one normal allele, usually don't exhibit any symptoms, but they can still pass on the faulty gene to their progeny.

Genetic Counselling and Testing

Through the identification of mutations in the XP-related genes, genetic testing can validate an XP diagnosis. For impacted families to comprehend the inheritance pattern, recurrence risks, and family planning consequences, genetic counseling is crucial. For families with a known history of XP, further options include prenatal and preimplantation genetic diagnosis.

Molecular Biology Advances Associated with XP

Molecular biology discoveries have greatly expanded our knowledge of XP:

A thorough examination of the XP genes for mutations is made possible by **Next-generation sequencing (NGS)**.

- **CRISPR/Cas9**: Gene editing potential to repair XP gene mutations.

- **Functional assays**: Evaluate the effect of particular mutations on the ability to repair DNA.

- **Model organisms**: Research on cell lines and mice sheds light on the pathophysiology and possible treatments.

Comprehending Genetic Propensity

Genetic susceptibility to XP entails knowledge of how particular mutations impact the operation of the NER pathway. Based on the kind and location of mutations, studies on genotype-phenotype correlations aid in the prediction of disease severity. Furthermore, variations in the XP gene may affect a person's vulnerability to UV-induced damage and their chance of developing skin cancer.

Future Paths for Genetic Research

Prospects for future investigation encompass:

Gene therapy: Research ways to fix or make up for XP genes that aren't working properly.

Medical strategies: Creating medications that boost NER activity that is still present or shield the body from UV rays.

- **Personalised medicine**: Developing preventative and therapeutic plans according to each patient's unique genetic profile.

- **Preventive strategies**: Population screening programs are used to identify and manage carriers.

In conclusion, deficiencies in the NER system, which result in an incapacity to repair UV-induced DNA damage, are at the core of the genetic and molecular underpinnings of XP. Gaining insight into these pathways is essential to enhancing XP patients' diagnosis, course of therapy, and, ultimately, quality of life. Research into novel strategies to lessen the effects of this difficult illness is still ongoing.

CHAPTER 3

DIAGNOSTICS AND CLINICAL SIGNS

Symptoms related to the skin

The rare hereditary condition known as xeroderma pigmentosum (XP) mainly affects the skin. When someone has XP, dermatological symptoms are frequently the first symptoms to be identified. Extreme sensitivity to sunlight, which results in severe sunburns even after little sun exposure, is how these symptoms appear. Especially on sun-exposed areas like the face, neck, and hands, this sensitivity can lead to dry, rough, and thicker skin over time, as well as the formation of freckle-like spots called lentigines. In extreme situations, people with XP may experience a markedly earlier onset of skin cancers than people in general, including melanoma, squamous cell carcinoma, and basal cell carcinoma.

Symptoms of Neurology

Additionally, XP affects the neural system, which in certain people results in neurological problems. Progressive cognitive decline, trouble balancing and coordinating, hearing loss, trouble speaking, and in certain situations, seizures, are some of these symptoms. The accumulation of DNA damage in nerve cells brought on by the incapacity to effectively repair ultraviolet (UV) light-induced DNA damage is the cause of the neurological symptoms associated with XP.

Symptoms of the Eyes

A distinguishing feature of XP is ocular involvement. People with XP may have dry eyes, irritated eyes, photophobia, or sensitivity to light. UV radiation exposure can cause corneal ulcers, conjunctivitis, and in extreme situations, keratitis, or clouding of the cornea, which can result in blindness.

XP's Progressive Nature

Since XP is a progressive disorder, symptoms usually get worse over time, especially after prolonged sun exposure. People with XP are more likely to acquire multiple skin malignancies and to experience severe neurological and ocular symptoms as the damage to their DNA increases.

Medical Requirements

Clinical signs, family history, and laboratory tests are used to diagnose XP. A history of severe sunburn with little sun exposure, numerous lentigines or freckle-like spots in sun-exposed areas, and a family history of XP or consanguinity (parents related by blood) are among the diagnostic factors. Assays for DNA repair may be used in lab tests to evaluate a cell's capacity to repair UV-induced DNA damage.

Diagnosis Differential

Proper management needs to differentiate XP from other illnesses that present with comparable symptoms. Other photosensitive conditions like

Cockayne syndrome, porphyrias, and solar urticaria are among the prominent differential diagnoses. Specialized diagnostic examinations and genetic tests aid in distinguishing XP from these disorders.

The Diagnostic Role of Dermatologists

Dermatologists are essential in the diagnosis of XP because they evaluate skin symptoms, do skin biopsies as required, and determine the likelihood of skin malignancies. Additionally, they provide sun protection measures and routine skin exams to patients and their families to detect early symptoms of skin cancer.

The Function of Ophthalmologists and Neurologists:

The comprehensive care of patients with XP involves the involvement of neurologists and ophthalmologists. Neurologists assess neurological symptoms, treat neurological problems, and do neuroimaging scans when necessary. Ophthalmologists diagnose and treat eye-related conditions, including early identification of ocular cancers, as well as evaluate ocular symptoms and conduct eye exams.

Biopsy and Imaging Methods:

Neurological problems, such as brain atrophy or abnormalities, can be evaluated in people with XP using imaging techniques like MRI and CT scans. To help in the diagnosis and treatment of XP, skin biopsies are carried out to assess skin lesions for the existence of skin malignancies or aberrant DNA repair pathways.

Gemological Testing Confirmatory:

Confirmatory genetic testing is necessary to detect particular gene mutations and confirm the diagnosis of XP. Examples of this testing include DNA sequencing of XP-related genes (e.g., XPA,

XPB, and XPC). To address the inheritance pattern of XP, possible risks for family members, and current management alternatives, such as sun protection techniques, routine tests, and experimental genetic medicines, genetic counseling is frequently advised.

CHAPTER 4

STRATEGIES FOR MANAGEMENT AND TREATMENT

Skincare and Sun Protection

A hereditary condition known as Xeroderma Pigmentosum (XP) causes the skin to be extremely sensitive to ultraviolet (UV) light. Taking care of your skin and avoiding the sun are essential parts of managing XP. This comprises:

- **UV Protection:** Using high SPF broad-spectrum sunscreen, donning hats, sunglasses, and protective apparel, as well as looking for shade during the hottest parts of the day.

- **Skin Care:** Avoiding harsh chemicals or abrasive exfoliants; moisturizing to prevent dryness and cracking; gentle cleansing procedures using light, non-irritating products.

Systemic and Topical Interventions

The following topical and systemic therapies can be used to address symptoms associated with XP:

- **Topical Treatments:** To control inflammation and lessen skin lesions, topical steroids or immunomodulators may be used.

- **Systemic Treatments:** To manage skin alterations and lower the risk of skin cancer, doctors may give systemic drugs such as retinoids.

Skin Lesion Surgical Options

Surgical methods including excision, cryotherapy, or Mohs surgery may be required for serious skin lesions or skin malignancies to remove damaged tissue while protecting healthy skin.

Handling Neurological Illnesses

Neurological problems may result from XP's impact on the nervous system. In addition to routine neurological examinations, management techniques may include medication to control seizures or other neurological problems.

Ophthalmological Procedures

Ophthalmologic therapies are necessary because UV radiation increases the risk of eye injury. This could entail getting frequent eye checkups, donning protective eyewear, and receiving treatment for ailments like ocular surface tumors or cataracts.

The Function of Dietary Supplements and Antioxidants

Dietary supplements and antioxidants may be helpful in the management of XP. They can promote general health and help combat oxidative damage brought on by UV exposure. However, a healthcare provider should be consulted regarding their unique responsibilities.

Emotional and Psychological Assistance

Emotionally, living with XP can be difficult. Counseling or support groups are examples of psychological support that can be helpful for people and families managing the effects of XP on everyday life and well-being.

Formulating a Complete Care Strategy

Coordination between multiple medical specialists, such as dermatologists, neurologists, ophthalmologists, and genetic counselors, is essential in a comprehensive care plan for XP patients. Sun protection, medicinal interventions, routine exams, and continuous monitoring should all be covered under this plan.

Clinical trials and emerging therapies

For XP, researchers are always looking for novel medicines and treatments. Enrolling in clinical trials can provide access to experimental medicines and further medical understanding of the management of XP.

Extended Monitoring and Follow-up

To manage XP, regular long-term follow-up and monitoring are essential. This involves routine evaluations of the skin, eyes, nervous system, and general health to identify and treat any changes or issues early on.

Through the integration of these tactics into an all-encompassing care plan, people with XP can maximize their quality of life, reduce problems, and remain up to date on the most recent advancements in XP management.

CHAPTER 5

XERODERMA PIGMENTOSUM: A DAY IN THE LIFE

Adaptations for Daily Life

To maintain safety and well-being, people with Xeroderma Pigmentosum (XP) need to make several adjustments to their daily routine. Among these modifications are:

1. **UV Protection:** People should limit their exposure to the sun by remaining inside during the hours of most sunshine and wearing high-SPF sunscreen, protective clothes, caps, and sunglasses. This is because XP is very susceptible to ultraviolet (UV) radiation.

2. **Indoor Environment:** You may lessen UV exposure by making your home a safe place to be by installing UV-blocking window films, and UV-

filtering lamps, and drawing your curtains throughout the day.

3. **Skin Care:** Maintaining the health of your skin requires consistent skincare regimens that include mild washing, moisturizing, and avoiding harsh chemicals or irritants.

4. **Eye Protection:** UV damage to the eyes can be prevented by wearing UV-blocking eyewear and making sure interior areas have enough illumination.

5. **Dietary Considerations:** Antioxidants and vitamins abundant in a well-balanced diet can promote general health and resilience of the skin.

Value of Regularity and Regularity

For someone with XP to effectively manage their illness, they must establish a consistent daily regimen. This comprises:

1. **UV-Free Zones:** Establishing areas where UV exposure is either limited or minimal at home and work is a good idea.

2. **Organised Activities:** Arranging outdoor pursuits for the early morning or late afternoon, when the sun's rays are at their lowest.

3. **Medication and Treatment:** Following prescription regimens and seeing doctors frequently to assess the condition of your skin and any possible problems.

4. **Sleep Hygiene:** Keeping a regular sleep routine and making sure your bedroom is dark and UV-free will help you sleep better and feel better overall.

Handling Social and Emotional Difficulties:

There are certain social and emotional difficulties associated with having XP, such as:

1. **Social Isolation:** People with XP may feel socially isolated since they must avoid sunshine.

Isolation can be lessened by promoting online social connections, enrolling in XP support groups, and educating loved ones about the illness.

2. **Emotional Well-Being:** Coping techniques that promote resilience and emotional well-being include mindfulness, counseling, and indoor hobbies and activities.

3. **Peer Support:** Using XP support networks to connect with people who have gone through similar situations can be a great way to get understanding and emotional support.

Educational Factors and Modifications

Educational concerns and accommodations are crucial for children with XP:

1. **UV-Safe Schools:** Creating UV-safe spaces, like covered outdoor areas and classrooms with

UV filters, in collaboration with schools guarantees a safer learning environment.

2. **Flexible Learning choices:** Providing homeschooling or online courses as flexible learning choices might help meet the demand for UV protection during the school day.

3. **Educational Support:** Educating instructors, students, and school personnel about XP through materials and resources promotes inclusivity and understanding.

Adjustments for Workplace and Employment

People with XP may need modifications at work to maintain productivity and safety:

1. **UV-Protected Workspace:** Reducing UV exposure is possible by setting up a UV-protected workspace with UV-filtering lights, window films, and sufficient shading.

2. **Flexible Work Arrangements:** People can minimize UV exposure during journeys by avoiding peak sunshine hours and opting for remote work choices.

3. **Educating Employers:** Offering UV protection equipment or modifying work schedules are examples of reasonable accommodations that can be discussed with employers to foster a positive work environment.

Activities for Leisure and Recreation

Despite obstacles, people with XP can engage in leisure activities as long as they take the right safety measures:

1. **Indoor Hobbies:** Reading, drawing, cooking, or playing an instrument are examples of indoor hobbies that promote creativity and relaxation.

2. **UV-Safe Outings:** Arranging activities that protect you from the sun, such as visits to

theatres, museums, or indoor sports facilities, is a great way to have fun.

3. **Adaptive Sports:** Getting involved in adaptive sports or UV-safe activities, including indoor swimming or UV-safe video games, promotes social connection and physical activity.

Community Resources and Support Networks

For people and families impacted by XP, establishing connections with support systems and making use of available community resources is essential:

1. **XP Support Groups:** Participating in online communities or support groups for XP offers a forum for exchanging experiences, getting access to resources, and getting emotional support.

2. **Medical Professionals:** Establishing a network of medical professionals with XP management experience guarantees all-encompassing care and prompt interventions.

3. **Community Programmes:** Taking part in fundraising events, educational workshops, and community programs helps spread the word about XP and cultivates community support.

Caring for an XP Child

Parents are essential in giving care and support to their children who have XP.

1. **UV Safety Education:** Teaching kids about UV safety precautions, such as donning sunscreen and protective clothes, helps them develop lifetime XP management skills.

2. **Advocacy:** Promoting UV-safe settings in educational institutions, parks, and public areas helps to guarantee children's inclusion and safety.

3. **Emotional Support:** Boosting resilience and coping mechanisms involves offering emotional support, being transparent in communication, and establishing connections

with other parents going through similar difficulties.

Stories and Experiences from Myself

Within the XP community, exchanging personal tales and encounters promotes empathy, camaraderie, and support:

1. **Narrative Sharing:** Communicating via blogs, social media, or support group meetings about one's experiences, struggles, and victories fosters empathy and understanding.

2. **Inspiration and Hope:** Learning about the tenacity and experiences of others gives one hope, drive, and a feeling of acceptance in the XP community.

Extended Perspective and Prognosis

Despite the difficulties associated with XP, improvements in medical research and UV protection technologies provide hope for better long-term results:

1. **Medical Advancements:** Continued research in photoprotection, genetics, and therapy alternatives may result in improvements in the management of XP and the quality of life.

2. **Lifestyle Management:** People with XP can effectively manage their illness and maximize long-term outcomes by following UV protection measures, scheduling regular healthcare visits, and leading a healthy lifestyle.

In summary, managing Xeroderma Pigmentosum necessitates a blend of pragmatic adjustments, psychological assistance, advocacy, and community involvement to guarantee security, health, and standard of living for those impacted by this uncommon hereditary disorder and their family.

CHAPTER 6

RISK REDUCTION AND PREVENTATIVE ACTIONS

UV Protection and Sun Safety

The hallmark of the hereditary condition Xeroderma Pigmentosum (XP) is a high sensitivity to ultraviolet (UV) radiation from sunshine. For people with XP, sun safety and UV protection are essential to preventing skin damage and lowering the chance of developing skin cancer. The following are important tactics:

1. **Sun Avoidance:** Avoid going outside when the sun is at its strongest, from 10 a.m. to 4 p.m.

2. **Seek Shade:** Remain in locations with shade or provide your own with canopies, hats, and umbrellas.

3. **Protective Clothes:** Put on dark, tightly woven clothing that covers your skin, such as

gloves, long sleeves, slacks, and sunglasses that filter UV rays.

4. **UV-Protective Gear:** Make use of UV-blocking umbrellas and caps with wide brims.

5. **Sunscreen**: After swimming or perspiring, and every two hours, use a broad-spectrum sunscreen with a high SPF (30 or above).

6. **UV Index Awareness: Plan outside activities based on the UV index, which you should check every day.

The Value of Regular Screening and Early Detection

Regular screening and early diagnosis of skin problems are essential for controlling XP. This is the reason why:

1. **Risk of Skin Cancer**: XP raises the possibility of getting skin cancer, including melanoma and non-melanoma types.

2. **Regular Skin Checks:** To ensure early detection of any abnormal skin lesions or changes, encourage regular skin self-examinations and dermatologist appointments.

3. **Diagnostic Tests:** To monitor skin health and identify any cancers early, use diagnostic tests including skin biopsies and imaging examinations.

Accessories and Clothes for Protection

A physical barrier against UV rays can be created by wearing appropriate clothing and accessories:

1. **Materials for Clothes:** Opt for apparel composed of UV-blocking materials or UV-protective fabrics.

2. **Hats and Gloves:** To protect the face, neck, and hands, wear broad-brimmed hats and UV-blocking gloves.

3. **Sunglasses:** To prevent UV damage to the eyes and surrounding skin, wear sunglasses with UV protection.

Environmental Safety Procedures

Establish a secure atmosphere to reduce UV exposure:

1. **Indoor Activities:** Promote indoor pursuits when the sun is at its strongest.

2. **Window Tinting:** To lessen UV ray penetration indoors, use UV-protective window coatings or tints.

3. **Artificial Lighting:** Make use of artificial lighting sources that emit the fewest UV rays.

Function of sunblocks and sunscreens

Sunblocks and sunscreens are necessary for UV protection:

1. **SPF Selection:** Use broad-spectrum, high SPF sunscreens to protect yourself from UVA and UVB radiation.

2. **Application:** Especially after swimming or perspiring, liberally apply sunscreen and reapply as needed.

3. **Use of Sunblock:** For extra protection, think about applying physical sunblocks with zinc oxide or titanium dioxide.

4 Steer Clear of Photosensitizing Agents

There are drugs, chemicals, and other substances that can make you more photosensitive:

1. **Medication Review:** Discuss medication reviews with medical professionals to detect photosensitizing substances and look into other possibilities.

2. **Chemical Exposure:** Reduce your exposure to substances that can aggravate photosensitivity, such as some scents and dyes.

Raising Awareness and Conducting Educational Campaigns

It's essential to run educational efforts and awareness initiatives to spread knowledge and encourage sun safety:

1. **Public Awareness:** Run educational efforts to increase public knowledge about UV protection, sun safety precautions, and XP.

2. **School Programmes:** Introduce sun safety initiatives in schools to inform parents, instructors, and students about the dangers of UV rays and how to avoid them.

3. **Community Outreach:** Assist people with XP and their families by collaborating with local groups and medical professionals to offer educational materials and support.

School and Community Involvement

Participation in the community and school can help create a supportive atmosphere for people with XP:

1. **Support Groups:** Create support groups so that people with XP and their families can exchange resources, knowledge, and experiences.

2. **School Policies:** Promote the implementation of sun safety measures in schools, such as shade structures, options for UV-protective apparel, and sun safety instruction.

3. **Peer Education:** Encourage pupils to encourage and educate one another to foster inclusivity for people with XP and sun safety practices.

Initiatives from the Government and Nonprofits

Governments and nonprofit groups are essential sources of funding for advocacy, support services, and research:

1. **Research Funding:** Encourage government-funded studies to improve our knowledge of XP and its prevention, treatment, and management.

2. **Advocacy Efforts:** Make the case for laws that advance sun safety, UV protection resource accessibility, and assistance for people with XP.

3. **Non-profit Support:** Work with nonprofit groups to offer monetary grants, educational resources, and community outreach initiatives to people with XP.

Prospective Routes for Prevention

Future developments in XP prevention are being shaped by ongoing research:

1. **Genetic Counselling:** To support educated decision-making and prompt intervention, provide genetic counseling and testing to individuals and families at risk of XP.

2. **Precision Medicine:** Examine individualized therapeutic modalities for XP patients, including gene therapy and targeted therapies.

3. **Public Health Initiatives:** To enhance early detection, diagnosis, and management of XP, allocate funds to public health campaigns, research projects, and healthcare facilities.

Despite their increased sensitivity to UV radiation, people with Xeroderma Pigmentosum can live healthier and more protected lives by putting these preventive measures and risk reduction methods into practice.

CHAPTER 7

STUDIES AND DEVELOPMENTS IN XP

Notable Achievers in XP Research

Important historical turning points in the study of Xeroderma pigmentosum (XP) have influenced our knowledge of this uncommon hereditary condition. Here are some significant turning points, from its first identification to ground-breaking discoveries:

1. **Discovery and Identification (1874–1882):** Moritz Kaposi published the first clinical reports of XP in 1874, and Hebra and Kaposi further characterized the condition in 1882.

2. **Sunlight Sensitivity Link (1940s-1950s):** Cleaver's research during the 1940s and 1950s helped to clarify the relationship between XP and sunlight sensitivity, as well as its function in DNA repair.

3. **DNA Repair Defect (1960s–1970s):** The identification of DNA repair errors in individuals with XP, especially by Dr. James Cleaver and others, represented a major advancement in our knowledge of the molecular causes of XP.

4. **Genetic Mapping (1980s-1990s):** During the 1980s and 1990s, advances in genetic mapping techniques made it easier to identify particular genes that cause XP, including XPA, XPC, and others.

5. **Gene Therapy Breakthrough (2010s):** New developments in gene therapy strategies for XP have emerged recently, providing encouraging paths for future therapies.

Genetic Research Breakthroughs

The identification of prospective treatment targets and the unraveling of underlying mechanisms in XP has been made possible by genetic research. Important discoveries consist of:

1. **Identification of XP Genes:** More than 20 genes have been linked to XP, offering information about the DNA repair pathways that are impacted in XP patients.

2. **Functional Characterization:** Thorough research has clarified the roles that XP-related genes play in genome maintenance and nucleotide excision repair (NER).

3. **Gene Editing Technologies:** New developments in gene editing techniques, such as CRISPR-Cas9, have the potential to fix genetic flaws in the cells of XP sufferers.

4. **Genomic Research**: Extensive genomic research has helped to clarify the genetic variety and phenotypic diversity seen in XP.

New Developments in Therapeutic Strategies

Innovative approaches to treating XP center on symptom management, averting complications, and investigating potential treatments. Important strategies consist of:

1. **Sun Protection:** To reduce UV-induced damage, XP patients must adhere to strict sun protection measures, such as wearing UV-blocking clothes, hats, and sunscreen.

2. **Topical Treatments:** The possibility of topical treatments, such as antioxidants and DNA repair enzymes, to repair UV-induced DNA damage is being investigated.

3. **Gene Therapy:** In an attempt to address genetic flaws in XP sufferers' cells, experimental gene therapy techniques may provide a treatment for the condition.

4. **Stem Cell Therapy:** Researchers are looking into the potential of stem cell-based treatments to regenerate injured tissues in XP patients.

Medical Studies and Trials

An essential part of assessing novel therapies and interventions for XP is clinical trial participation. Important features of research and clinical trials include:

1. **Experimental Therapies:** Clinical trials assess the effectiveness and safety of experimental treatments in individuals with XP, including stem cell transplantation and gene therapy.

2. **Longitudinal research:** Long-term research evaluates how XP symptoms develop, how well treatments work, and how well impacted people's quality of life is.

3. **Collaborative Research:** Strong data gathering and analysis are made possible by multicenter collaborations, which enable large-scale clinical trials.

4. **Patient engagement:** Increasing therapy options and advancing XP research require patient engagement in clinical studies.

Interactions Between Research Organisations

To expedite XP research and turn results into clinical applications, research institutions must work together. Important components of teamwork include:

1. **Data Sharing:** By encouraging cooperation and data sharing, collaborative projects make it easier for researchers to access a variety of datasets.

2. **Interdisciplinary Teams:** To address the complicated nature of XP, multidisciplinary teams including geneticists, dermatologists, oncologists, and molecular biologists work together.

3. **International Partnerships:** International collaborations promote the sharing of resources, the exchange of expertise, and cooperative research projects to improve XP research worldwide.

Patient Advocacy Groups' Role

Patient advocacy groups are essential for promoting research efforts, helping patients and their families, and increasing public awareness. Advocacy groups play important roles in the following areas:

1. **Awareness Campaigns:** Campaigns to increase public knowledge about XP, its symptoms, and the value of sun protection are carried out by advocacy groups.

2. **Support Services:** They offer financial aid, educational materials, counseling, and other forms of support to XP patients and their families.

3. **Funds for Research:** Advocacy organizations frequently provide funds for studies, support clinical trials, and push for more institutional and governmental support for XP research.

XP Research Funding & Grants

Grants and funding are crucial for maintaining XP research initiatives and encouraging creativity in the area. Important financing sources consist of:

1. **Government funds:** XP research initiatives are supported by funds from government organizations such as the National Science Foundation (NSF) and the National Institutes of Health (NIH).

2. **Philanthropic Organisations:** Grants and financial support for XP research activities are provided by non-profit organizations and foundations, including the XP Family Support Group and the XP Society.

3. **Industry Partnerships:** Funding for translational research and clinical trials in XP is made possible by partnerships with biotech and pharmaceutical businesses.

Journals and Scientific Publications

The dissemination of XP research discoveries and the promotion of scientific discourse are greatly aided by scientific publications and journals. Important books and periodicals consist of:

1. **Journal of Investigative Dermatology:** Research on skin conditions, including XP, is published in this journal. It addresses issues including molecular mechanisms, therapeutic modalities, and patient outcomes.

2. **Genes & Development:** Research on gene expression, DNA repair pathways, and genetic abnormalities are published in this journal, offering insights into the molecular pathways associated with XP.

3. **Nature Reviews Cancer:** Papers in this journal address a variety of cancer-related subjects, such as UV-induced DNA damage, skin cancer risk in individuals with XP, and new treatment options.

Routines for Future Research

Subsequent studies in XP are well-positioned to tackle significant obstacles and investigate inventive approaches. Among the promising avenues for investigation are:

1. **Precision Medicine Approaches:** Personalised treatments based on unique genetic profiles have the potential to maximize therapeutic benefits while reducing side effects.

2. **Targeted Therapies:** One possible therapy approach is to focus on particular molecular pathways, like NER deficiencies, that are involved in the pathophysiology of XP.

3. **Regenerative Medicine:** New methods of treating skin damage caused by XP may result from developments in regenerative medicine, such as tissue engineering and stem cell-based therapy.

4. **Gene Editing Technologies:** As gene editing techniques like base editing and epigenome editing continue to progress, they may provide accurate and focused therapies to fix genetic flaws in XP.

Impact of Patient Care Research

The following areas of XP research have had a significant impact on patient care:

1. **Enhanced Diagnosis**: Early detection and treatments are now possible due to enhanced diagnostic accuracy brought about by a better understanding of XP genetics and biomarkers.

2. **Personalised Treatment Plans:** Based on patient needs and genetic profiles, customized

treatment plans have been made possible by research-driven insights.

3. **Enhanced Quality of Life:** XP patients and their families now enjoy an enhanced quality of life thanks to cutting-edge therapies, supportive care services, and community resources.

CHAPTER 8

ADVOCACY AND SUPPORT NETWORKS

The Function of Organisations and Support Groups

Support groups and organizations are essential in helping people with Xeroderma Pigmentosum (XP) and their families by offering resources and assistance. These clubs provide possibilities for networking with people going through similar struggles, as well as emotional support and education about the illness. They frequently plan social activities, seminars, and meetings to help XP sufferers and their families feel more connected to one another.

Medical and Social Service Access

People with XP need to have access to social and medical assistance to effectively manage their disease. Monitoring and treatment, entail routine visits to dermatologists and other specialists. Home care, transportation aid, and access to community support programs are examples of social services. To guarantee complete treatment, patients and their families must understand the services that are available and how to access them.

Legal Advocacy and Rights

It is essential that people with XP are aware of their legal rights and actively fight for them. This covers rights to work, education, healthcare, and accessibility. Working with legislators, governmental organizations, and agencies to advance laws that help XP patients—like financing for research, availability of specialized care, and accommodations in different contexts—may be a part of advocacy activities.

Financial Support and Insurance

Because XP is so expensive to treat, it can be difficult for affected persons to navigate insurance coverage and apply for financial aid. Organizations and support groups frequently offer advice on how to access financial aid programs, appeal denials, and comprehend insurance coverage. This can entail paying for prescription drugs, medical supplies, and other essential expenditures.

Psychological and Counselling Services

It is imperative to seek counseling and mental health assistance to treat the psychological and emotional effects of having XP. Patients and their loved ones may benefit from individual therapy, support groups, and family counseling to help them deal with stress, anxiety, and other mental health issues. The availability of mental health providers who are aware of the particular difficulties faced by XP can have a major impact on general well-being.

Workshops & Seminars for Education

Important information regarding XP, its management, and other subjects like sun protection, skincare, and genetic counseling can be found in informative courses and seminars. These gatherings can be planned by advocacy groups, support groups, or medical professionals to equip families and patients with the information and abilities needed to successfully manage life with XP.

Community Development and Networking

Through networking and community-building events, families and patients with XP can connect with others who have gone through similar things. Online discussion boards, social media groups, and in-person meetings led by organizations and support groups can all be used for this. Creating a network of people who support you can provide you with a sense of community, practical guidance, and emotional validation.

History of Patients and Families

Narratives from patients and their families are potent resources for educating the public about XP and motivating members of society. Public speaking, films, or written accounts of personal experiences can all be used to educate the public, lessen stigma, and promote empathy and understanding. Those going through comparable struggles can also find inspiration and hope in these tales.

Input from Donors and Volunteers

The efforts of organizations devoted to XP campaigning and support are greatly aided by volunteer and donation contributions. Volunteers might lend their time and expertise to peer support, event planning, or awareness-raising initiatives. Contributions ensure ongoing support and advancement in the field by helping to finance programs, services, and research that aid XP sufferers and their families.

Effective Advocacy Strategies

Persistence, teamwork, and strategic preparation are necessary for effective XP advocacy. This could consist of:

1. **Creating Alliances:** To increase advocacy efforts, forming alliances with researchers, policymakers, healthcare providers, and community leaders.

2. **Raising Awareness:** Informing the public, media, and decision-makers about the effects of XP, the resources that are required, and its implications.

3. **Policy Advocacy:** Promoting laws that give financing for research, healthcare access,

disability rights, and public accommodations for people with XP top priority.

4. **Community Engagement:** Using digital platforms, events, and outreach to interact with the XP community to disseminate information and rally support.

5. **Empowering People:** Giving people with XP and their families the tools they need to stand up for what's right, get resources, and take part in life-altering decision-making.

Advocacy initiatives can significantly improve the lives of Xeroderma Pigmentosum-affected persons and their families by utilizing these tactics.

CHAPTER 9
CASE STUDIES AND ACTUAL INSTANCES

Early-Onset XP Case Study

People who experience the signs of Xeroderma Pigmentosum (XP) early in life—typically in infancy or early childhood—are referred to as early onset XP patients. Typically, this case study entails a thorough investigation of the clinical presentation, hereditary variables, contextual circumstances, and difficulties that patients and their families encounter. It might draw attention to the symptoms' quick development, heightened vulnerability to UV rays, and the necessity of taking precautions against the sun at a very young age.

Case Study: XP With Late-Onset

As opposed to Early-Onset XP, Late-Onset XP typically manifests its symptoms later in life, in adolescence or maturity. This case study explores the distinctive features of XP onset later in life, such as possible differences in clinical presentations, difficulties in diagnosing the condition because of the delayed onset, and effects on lifestyle and career decisions.

Examining Case: Neurological Issues

In certain instances, XP has been linked to neurological problems including hearing loss, cognitive impairment, and neurological degeneration. This case study investigates the particular neurological manifestations, how they develop over time, and the management techniques used to deal with these issues. These techniques may entail a multidisciplinary approach integrating rehabilitative medicine, neurology, and genetics.

Case Study: Effective Treatment Strategies

This case study highlights effective XP treatment approaches and interventions, such as genetic counseling, photoprotection strategies, skin cancer screenings, and cutting-edge treatments like stem cell or gene therapy. It focuses on situations when prompt diagnosis and all-encompassing care have greatly enhanced patient outcomes and quality of life.

Case Study: Diagnostic Difficulties

Because XP is uncommon, presents differently, and overlaps with other genetic and dermatological diseases, diagnosing it can be difficult. This case study looks at the typical diagnostic challenges that medical professionals deal with, like delayed diagnosis, complicated genetic testing, and the significance of clinical suspicion in quickly identifying people with XP.

Case Study: Family Effects

XP has a significant effect on the afflicted person as well as their family, who frequently assume a critical role in supporting and managing the disease. This case study explores the logistical, financial, and emotional obstacles that XP families must overcome. These obstacles include decisions on genetic counseling, carer duties, and adjusting to the unknowns associated with a chronic genetic disorder.

Case Study: Aspects Psychosocial

Significant psychological effects of having XP can include social isolation, anxiety, depression, and problems with body image. In this case study, the psychosocial difficulties that XP patients face are examined, along with their coping strategies, peer support systems, and the role that mental health providers have in providing these components of care.

Example Study: Prolonged Administration

The long-term care of XP entails neurodevelopmental evaluations, UV protection techniques, continuous skin cancer screening, and attending to patients' changing needs as they mature. This case study demonstrates effective long-term care strategies, such as follow-up appointments, patient education, and the use of adaptive technology to improve independence and quality of life.

Intellectual Gains from Case Studies

Examining different XP case cases teaches researchers, policymakers, and medical professionals important lessons. The significance of early diagnosis, individualized treatment plans, interdisciplinary teamwork, patient and family education, and the ongoing search for cutting-edge treatments and supportive services are a few examples of these teachings.

Repercussions for Upcoming Procedures

The application of learnings from XP case studies to dermatology, genetics, neurology, and oncology guides future procedures. To fully understand the intricacies of XP pathophysiology and therapy, it emphasizes the need for enhanced diagnostic tools, increased accessibility to genetic testing, targeted medicines based on specific XP subtypes, patient rights advocacy, support services, and continued research.

CHAPTER 10

PUBLIC AWARENESS, EDUCATION, AND ADVOCACY

The Value of Spreading Knowledge About XP

Extreme sensitivity to ultraviolet (UV) light is a characteristic of the rare genetic condition known as XP. Increasing awareness is crucial because it facilitates:

Early Diagnosis: Better patient outcomes can result from early diagnosis and intervention due to increased awareness.

- **Preventative Measures**: Sunlight and UV exposure should be avoided by those who have XP. Public awareness campaigns can inform people of the value of taking precautions such as using sunscreen, dressing in protective gear, and remaining inside during the sun's strongest hours.

- **Community Support**: Raising awareness creates networks of support within the community, which lessens isolation and offers patients and their families both practical and emotional assistance.

Health Care Professional Education Programmes

Programs of education aimed at medical professionals are essential for:

Early Recognition: Educating medical professionals on how to identify XP symptoms will help them diagnose patients quickly and treat them appropriately.

Optimal Care: Ensuring that patients receive the greatest care and assistance possible is made possible by educating medical personnel about protocols particular to XP.

Campaigns for Patient Advocacy and Empowerment

Giving XP patients more authority entails:

- **Education**: Giving patients thorough knowledge about XP enables them to make wise decisions regarding their well-being.

Advocacy: Campaigns to promote patient rights, healthcare access, and the necessity of financing for research can be launched.

The Function of Digital Platforms and Social Media

Digital platforms are essential because they:

- **Amplifying Awareness**: Social media campaigns can disseminate factual information about XP and debunk falsehoods to a larger audience.

- **Building Communities**: Virtual communities offer a forum for XP patients, carers, and advocates to interact, exchange stories, and offer mutual support.

Advocating for Rare Diseases in Public Policy

Promoting public policies that assist rare diseases like XP entails:

Funding for Research: Encouraging more money to be allocated to XP research will hasten scientific progress and enhance patient outcomes.

- **Access to Treatment**: It is critical to support laws that guarantee people with rare diseases access to specialized medical care and therapies.

Interacting with Influencers and the Media

Participation in the media is essential for:

- **Awareness Campaigns**: By working with influencers and media sources, awareness campaigns can be amplified and reach a larger audience.

- **Storytelling**: By sharing the intimate tales of XP sufferers and supporters, we can humanize the illness and inspire compassion and understanding.

Events and Programmes for Community Outreach

Initiatives for community outreach can:

- **Educate**: Holding educational activities helps patients and their families by increasing awareness and offering support.

- **Support Collaboration**: Working together with businesses, organizations, and communities in the area can help XP patients establish a network of support.

Partnerships with Colleges and Universities

Benefits of interacting with educational institutions include:

- **Education and Training**: Raising awareness and comprehension is facilitated by integrating

XP education into healthcare training programs and school curricula.

- **Research Collaborations**: By collaborating with academic institutions, research on XP is advanced, leading to more possibilities for therapy.

Encouraging Accessibility and Inclusivity

Keeping accessibility and inclusivity in mind entails:

Accessible Information: Information that is available in a variety of formats, such as audio, braille, or different languages, guarantees accessibility for a range of demographics.

Inclusive Policies: Supporting inclusive policies in public areas, healthcare, and education advances the rights and welfare of XP patients.

Advocacy Activities' Effect on XP Research and Care

A significant influence of advocacy work is achieved by:

Financing for Research: Raising awareness of XP can result in increased financing for research, which in turn spurs advancements in management, diagnosis, and treatment.

- **Improved Care Standards**: By influencing healthcare standards and policies, advocacy can help XP patients receive better care and support.

All things considered, improving the lives of those who have Xeroderma Pigmentosum and advancing research and care in this area require a thorough commitment to advocacy, education, and public awareness.